W9-CKC-458

Joyce W. Hopp, R.N., M.P.H., Ph.D.

BABIES IN HER SADDLEBAGS

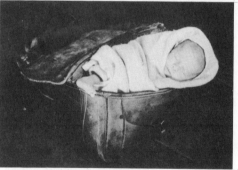

The mountain people of Kentucky and Tennessee have a tradition that babies arrive in saddlebags, similar to the more widely accepted tradition that babies are brought by storks.

Pacific Press Publishing Association
Boise, Idaho
Montemorelos, Nuevo Leon, Mexico
Oshawa, Ontario, Canada

Edited by Marvin Moore
Designed by Tim Larson
Cover by Lars Justinen
Type set in 10/12 Century Schoolbook

Library of Congress Cataloging in Publication Data

Hopp, Joyce W., 1927-
  Babies in her saddlebags.

  Bibliography: pp. 80, 81
  1. Lester, Betty. 2. Midwives—Great Britain—Biography. 3. Midwives—Kentucky—Biography. I. Title.
RG950.L47H67   1986   618.2'0233   [B]   86-20478

ISBN 0-8163-0677-X

Preface

The Frontier Nursing Service of Kentucky has been a romantic legend for nurses in the United States for over half a century. Ernest Poole's *Nurses on Horseback,* published in 1931, excited student nurses throughout the country. My nursing classmates and I were among those who caught the fervor in the years following World War II. We were all going to Kentucky! None of us ever did, but the memory remained. I would meet graduates of the service in East Africa, in India, in California.

Then, while I was on a speaking engagement at the hospital in Manchester, Kentucky, one of my former students offered me an opportunity to visit the headquarters of the Frontier Nursing Service in nearby Hyden. I jumped at the chance. We went to Wendover to join the regular staff for supper, then sat in the comfortable living room of the "Big House" as we listened to two of the nurse midwives trace the history of the FNS.

Betty Lester had worked until her retirement in 1971; Molly Lee was still actively working as a midwife. Their stories kept us up until a late hour, and even then we didn't want them to stop. I remarked, "Betty, you need to write those stories."

Betty laughed, and replied, "Oh, I will someday."

The next day as I was jogging around the track at Manchester, I got to thinking. "She will never write. She's eighty-five, and she'll just keep saying that. I wonder if she'd let me write it for her?"

Betty readily agreed, but when the time came a year later to actually sit down and tell her stories to me, she was very reluctant. She admitted she had hoped I wouldn't come back! For Betty is a modest person. What she has done, anyone could have done, she says. But it takes a certain stick-to-itiveness to give your whole life in an out-of-the-way place like Leslie County, Kentucky, and the ability to work cross-culturally that many do not possess. The hours of interviews Betty finally permitted form the basis for this book.

I conducted supplemental research, using the quarterly bulletins which the service has published since its inception. As I sat in the living room at Wendover, alone with the bulletins and my thoughts, I felt a sense of awe at the history I was privileged to be seeing firsthand. The founder's library volumes still fill the bookshelves. The worn furniture, the polished staircase, the stone fireplace all give the past a sense of currency, as though any moment you expect the place to be filled with nurses as they gather for afternoon tea.

This book has been written in the hope that it will bring the inspiration of nurse-midwifery alive today, that there are still nurses who will respond to that call. It was for that reason Betty allowed me to write her story.

Joyce Hopp
Loma Linda, California
August 1985

Acknowledgements

Claire Warner, the health education director at the Manchester Hospital, made my first contact with the Frontier Nursing Service possible. Betty Childers, nurse anesthetist at the Mary Breckinridge Hospital in Hyden, and her roommate, Charleine Beatty, shared their home on Thousandsticks Mountain; they fed and housed me during the time of my on-site research.

David Hatfield, administrator of the hospital, made all the historical facilities available: copies of early movies, recent video tapes, maps, and publications. Gabrielle Beasley searched for original copies of old photographs. Ruth Beeman, dean and director of the Frontier School of Midwifery and Family Nursing, provided information on the status of nurse-midwifery today.

Members of the Loma Linda University faculty, Ruth White and Roberta Moore, provided valuable assistance. Roberta, recently retired from her position as professor of journalism, read and reread portions of the manuscript as it emerged. Ruth, a nurse-midwife in addition to her position as director of the doctoral program in public health, furnished an international perspective on nurse-midwifery.

My husband, Kenneth, accepted with equanimity the absences the research for this book entailed and evinced interest even though nurse-midwifery is far removed from his profession of law.

But without Betty Lester, whose ready laughter and quick wit I have enjoyed as we worked together, this would have been a tedious undertaking. She made it fun!

JWH

Contents

Kentucky Midwife   9
Sawmill Explosion   17
Six Babies in Five Nights   24
Hants   29
No Guns Allowed   34
Floodtides   40
Varmints   46
The War in England   51
Help for Taronda   57
From Horses to Jeeps   62
Betty's Babies   69
Honors for the General   75
Epilogue   79
Photo Section   82

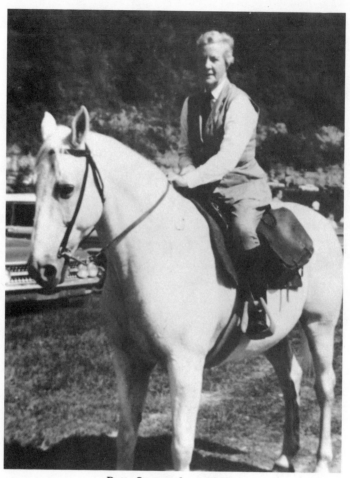

Betty Lester about 1960.

Kentucky Midwife

Betty looked across the muddy morass that was the main street of Hyden, Kentucky (population, 300). Was this really the place of which she had heard so much, the headquarters of the Frontier Nursing Service? The clapboard buildings that housed the bank and general store didn't look like they could serve as the headquarters of anything!

"Where's the hospital?" she asked her guide. "They told me they had just built a new hospital." But where, in this sparse settlement, was even one new building?

The courier pointed up the hill. There, high on the side of Thousandsticks Mountain overlooking the valley, was the hospital. It had been dedicated just a few days before and was even yet not completed.

Why was Betty Lester here? An English nurse-midwife, she had been recruited by Mary Breckinridge for the Frontier Nursing Service. Mrs. Breckinridge had chosen Leslie County, of which Hyden was the county seat, to initiate her project of trained nurse-midwives to serve rural families who were in desperate need of such care. The idea of nurses trained as midwives was novel in the United States in 1925. Until then, the women of the hill country had to rely on the "granny midwife" who chose the calling, but had no training for it.

Great Britain had trained nurses in midwifery for over fifty years. It was to this source Mary Breckinridge turned for her first nurses. She herself studied midwifery at the top-ranked British Hospital for Mothers and Babies in London. The Fron-

9

tier Nursing Service Mrs. Breckinridge started was a partner-
ship between the old country and the new. It would become
world famous. Sixty years later, it could boast that it had delivered over 20,000 babies with a loss of only eleven mothers.

But those accomplishments were only visionary that hot July
day in 1928. Betty was the last of five nurses to arrive that
summer. Two weeks of seasickness on the ocean voyage from
London, a hot train ride from New York, and a final plunge by
horseback deep into the hills of southeastern Kentucky had
brought her to Hyden.

"Well, you've made it," came the cheery greeting from the
chief nurse as Betty and her guide rode up to the hospital. And
who should it be but "Al" Logan, the American nurse with
whom Betty had studied in England the year before. How nice
for Al to be the first to welcome her! It was Al's book of photographs that had first sparked Betty's interest in joining the
Frontier Nursing Service. The album, left lying enticingly in
the nurses' quarters in London, had pictures of nurses on horseback—nurses who went to deliver babies in the homes of the
mountaineers in Kentucky.

"What an exciting life," Betty had exclaimed. "I've always
loved horses and dogs and babies and people. That place sounds
like it has them all."

"It has," Al assured her.

Now Betty was face to face with her choice, an adventure
that was to last over fifty years. Little did Betty realize that the
horses, the dogs, and the new babies would all become part of
her family. But that was in a future she could not see now. All
she could feel was the oppressive heat as Al showed her to her
room. No such thing as air conditioning. While the hospital did
own a generator for electricity, its use was limited to patient
service.

"Are you already to start work in the morning?" Al asked.
"You're to be assigned to this district. We've not had a nurse
working out of here, so you'll be starting new work."

Betty had one week with a nurse in another district to learn
the routine. Then she was on her own. She learned that each
nurse at the district outpost centers covered an area five miles

in each direction from her center. Betty's "center" was the hospital itself. The horseback trail to her district led up and over Thousandsticks Mountain and down to Bull Creek.

Four miles from Hyden, up the Middle Fork of the Kentucky, was Wendover, the home of Mary Breckinridge, the famous woman of whom she had heard so much. This daughter of a famous family had chosen to devote her life and her energies to saving the lives of mothers and babies in the hills of Kentucky. Her grandfather had been vice president of the United States; her father served as minister to Russia. Mary's was to be a demonstration project for rural areas, one which could be replicated in other parts of the world where physicians were scarce. As she was quick to point out, more American women had lost their lives bearing children than all the men who died in the wars the United States had fought since the Revolution. She would show that that picture could be changed!

Betty rode horseback up the river, across Muncy's Ford, and arrived at the "Big House," as the three-story log structure was dubbed. From this homey fortress, Mary Breckinridge directed the creation of the Frontier Nursing Service. And she was everything Betty had been led to expect.

"Come right in, my dear. Tell me about your trip," Mrs. Breckinridge invited. Betty found herself telling how she had always wanted to be a nurse, but that she had planned to use that nursing in India, not Kentucky!

"What brought you here instead?" Mrs. Breckinridge queried.

"The challenge of what you were trying to do," Betty responded. "I've always loved people, and these people sounded like they needed me, needed the kinds of things I can do."

"Yes, they need you. You're well prepared for this work. The matron at York Road [Lying-in Hospital, London] knows what I need here—nurses who can work on their own, with a physician as backup only for the most difficult cases." Mrs. Breckinridge went on to describe the lives her nurses were leading as they worked in lonely outpost centers. No telephones to call for help when they needed it. Only a man riding muleback over the rough trails.

"Can you ride? Yes, I know you came in by horseback from the end of the rail line. But how well can you ride?" Mrs. Breckinridge put the question to Betty that she had learned to ask each of her new nurses.

"I rode a lot when I was a girl," Betty replied. "I was brought up in the country. Farm horses mostly. We didn't own any horses, but the boys saw to it that I learned to ride."

"Good. We have horses at each of the centers, several here at Wendover, and some at the barn over at the hospital. Most of them come from down in the Bluegrass, especially chosen for our needs. They have to have a good gait, you know, or they will break all the bottles in your saddle bags!"

"And you must have a dog." With that, she presented Betty with a little collie pup. Since every one of the five new nurses that spring had received a similar gift, there was only the runt of the litter left by this time. The pup's tawny coat suggested a name, and Ginger it became on the spot.

Ginger was soon joined by a horse: "The Old Gray Mare." While the nurses didn't actually own their horses, they had their favorites which they most often rode. The Old Gray Mare quickly became Betty's favorite. The horse was indestructible, having served as a moonshiner's horse previously, and even yet carrying a bullet in her right hip. Betty soon discovered that her horse knew every trail, every creek, and nearly every boulder in Leslie County. She was a fine friend to have on the dark nights she was out delivering babies.

She had the horse and the dog. Now for the people. One of the nurses showed her around the area that was to be her district, introducing her to the families as they visited in homes up and down the creeks. Then Betty was on her own. She held clinic days regularly, both at the hospital and at different locations throughout her district. She invited the families to her clinics.

"They couldn't understand me, and I couldn't understand them," she recalls. "Some of the expressions they used, I simply didn't understand." The communication barrier between the British accent and the Kentucky dialect was quickly apparent. One of the most perplexing expressions was their response when she invited them to attend her clinics.

"I wouldn't care to," they would say. Then they would show up, and Betty wondered what happened. Gradually, she came to realize they meant that it would be no bother to come and that, indeed, they would do so.

Betty loved people and waited with longing to be accepted into this community. She didn't realize that the traditional attitude of the mountain people was to wait until "brought-on" people went away, that they were quite insular and rarely accepted people "from outside." So she sat on their porches, and she talked—but she got few answers.

"I don't think I'm going to make a success of this," Betty mourned to Al after a month of this noncommunication.

"Why not?"

"I can't get them to talk to me."

"Well," Al pointed out, "you don't expect them to throw their arms around your neck and be so friendly the first time they see you, do you?"

"No, but I wish they would say something to me sometimes," Betty rejoined.

A few weeks later, Al stopped Betty. "I've got something to tell you. One of your men from Bull Creek came over here today. He knows all the people in your area. I asked him, just for fun, 'How do you like your new nurse?'

" 'Well, we like her fine, but she sure is the talkingest woman I ever heard!' " he replied.

After that, Betty went on talking, knowing that they liked her, even if they didn't answer. Gradually, her talking brought a response. They talked about their families, their religion, their gardens. Some even volunteered information on how to make moonshine.

"I never used that information!" Betty says now. "And I always avoided politics. I don't know anything about politics, and never did! So I steered clear of that."

The picturesque expressions they used became part of her speech, although the precise British accent never disappeared. The twilight hour was always called "edge of dark," a time Betty enjoyed, although there were no sunsets to watch in the mountains.

In Hyden, Kentucky's back woods people, Betty found a home and a family—a very big family. She had lost both her mother and father before she was nineteen, so this family meant more to her than to those nurses who had families "on the outside."

The midwifery course at York Road Lying-in Hospital, the extra six months post-graduate training that the matron insisted on when she heard where Betty wanted to go—all Betty's training had been for this, the care of mothers and their babies. "You'll be on your own, you know."

"No doctor right around the corner," the matron had warned. Those words came vividly to her mind one night six months after she arrived in Hyden. "Heavens! What a night! We can all go to bed to sleep tonight, girls; no one can possibly come out on a night like this," Betty had exclaimed to her friends. One needs to live in the Kentucky mountains in order to understand just how truly the heavens can open up.

No sooner had Betty gotten the words out of her mouth, however, than she heard the familiar call outside, "Hallo-oo-oo."

"Oh, no!" Well, perhaps it would be a "primip" (one who was having her first baby), and thus she could delay going, since first babies usually took longer to arrive. No such luck!

"My wife's punishing awful bad. Need you in a hurry!" Lem exclaimed, the light of the hurricane lantern sending streaks of light across his wet face.

"I'll be ready in a moment." Betty slipped into her riding uniform, quickly lacing up her boots. Grabbing the midwifery bags, always kept packed and ready for just such a call, she headed for the barn and her horse.

The night was awful. Wind whipped through the trees, sending some crashing into the forest. The trail over Thousandsticks Mountain never seemed longer nor more slippery. A torrent of water washed down the trail, pushing rocks and brush ahead of it. The lantern Lem carried bobbed up and down crazily as his horse pressed forward ahead of her.

"Dear Lord, help me. I'll never make it on my own." Betty breathed the silent prayer over and over.

She recognized the fork in the trail where they turned up another creek. Here they had to ride right up the creek, as the water had risen and now covered the trail. Thank heaven for a horse that knew the way and was mighty careful where she put her feet. Betty reached out a hand and gave the Old Gray Mare a reassuring pat, then hastily drew it back under the protection of her rain cape.

But the rush through the night wasn't quite fast enough. Betty heard the baby's first cry as her feet touched the porch. Hurriedly, she spread out the contents of her midwifery bags and cut the cord. The placenta came immediately after, and with it a sudden gush of blood. Post-partum hemorrhage!

Quickly Betty massaged the mother's abdomen in an attempt to get the uterus to contract and shut off the flow of blood. Her brain whirled as she called to mind the next steps she had been trained to use.

Hypodermic injection of Pitocin. Keep massaging the uterus with one hand, give a dose of Ergotrate to the patient by mouth at the same time.

"I could use a couple more hands," she said to herself. She became aware that the woman's sister was standing in the doorway, watching with keen eyes every move Betty made.

"Help me lift the foot of the bed up on this chair," Betty said. "And extra blankets. Can you get me a couple?"

The room was chilly, but the perspiration stood out on Betty's forehead as she struggled to bring the hemorrhage and conse- quent shock under control.

Keep massaging the uterus. Check on the flow of blood. It's slowing!

Much more quickly than Betty dreamed possible, her patient came around. The pulse steadied and slowed, her lips became pink. The emergency was past. Betty's eyes met those of the sister. Had she, too, realized the gravity of the situation?

Betty waited until dawn, when she checked one more time for bleeding. Everything was normal. She started down the mountain trail. The rushing creeks had receded as quickly as they had risen, and all was peaceful as she headed back to the hospital.

Betty sat at her desk that morning, completing the routine paperwork, reporting the delivery. She filled in the facts: estimated hemorrhage, forty-eight ounces. Nearly three pints. But how could she write of her feelings as she heard the drip, drip, drip of the blood, dropping from the rubber sheet to the floor? Was this a life saved?

Evidently the women of the hills thought so. On her next visit, one of them remarked, "If it warn't for the nurses, I declare, I don't know what the women in this country would do."

The men noticed and appreciated too. Years after the frontier nurses had established centers and clinics throughout the hill country, one father remembered his heartbreak at the loss of his wife and baby in the year 1912. The woman in attendance was a seventy-five-year-old granny midwife. She did not always lose her patients, but she had not been trained, and when an emergency occurred she did not know what to do.

"I axed my mother, What would the people do when them old granny wimmin died out—there weren't many left," he recalled. "And she told me they'd be maybe a better way provided than them old wimmin. And when the nurses came thirteen years after that I remembered what she said." He and many other fathers had their wives and children alive because of the work of those nurses.

Betty had shown that she could deliver babies under difficult circumstances and bring the mother through alive. But what of the other disasters that happened in the mountains?

Sawmill Explosion

"You know, Miss Lester, we had ought to have a clinic of our own over here," Liza said one morning as Betty was doing her rounds in the Bull Creek District.

"Yes, that would be very nice. But the service has no money to put up any more buildings," Betty pointed out.

"Oh, we could all help. The menfolk around here could build it," Liza replied.

The remark started Betty thinking as her horse trotted along the trail later that morning. She had been using one room in the school teacher's house for her clinic each Thursday. It was nice of the teacher to lend her a room, but it didn't provide much privacy when she wanted to talk to a patient alone, and there was no waiting room in bad weather. People enjoyed visiting on the porch in the sunshine, but not when the rains came pouring down!

"Charlie, do you think the people around here would build me a clinic?" Betty tried the idea out on the teacher. He'd taught in the area for several years and knew the mountain people better than she did.

"Well, I sure do, Miss Lester," Charlie said, and he looked at his wife, Edith. "Not that we mind having you use our house, but it would be good if you could have your own place."

"Charlie could call a meeting at the school house," Edith said. "See what the folks think about it."

So plans were laid. Betty could hardly wait. Her very own clinic! She had rather envied Miss Peacock and Miss Williford,

17

the two nurses who had been constructing centers for the service. They had supervised the construction without ever having done any building before. If they could learn, so could she!

The schoolhouse was full that evening. "It looks like everyone in the area has come," she thought. "Charlie must have done a good job of advertising." The conversation ceased when he rose to speak.

"Now you all know Miss Lester has been coming over that mountain every week to hold a clinic for us," Charlie began. "We're mighty glad we have our own nurse, because most of you remember what it was like before the nurses came."

Heads nodded all around the room. Most of the younger children in the room had been delivered by the service nurses. Some of them might not be alive were it not for those nurses.

"Now Miss Lester needs our help," Charlie said. "She needs her own clinic here, a place where she can leave her equipment, where she can see the mamas and their babies every week. I thought if you knew what she needed, you all might help her get it. I think we could build her a clinic, don't you?" Charlie looked around the room.

There were a few moments of silence. "Wasn't anyone going to say anything?" Betty wondered. "Oh, dear."

But mountain people are careful thinkers and slow talkers. After what seemed like an eternity, but was probably only two minutes, one of the men spoke up. "Sure, we can help Miss Lester. We'll build her a clinic. Where does she want it?"

Charlie pointed out the window. "I thought we could put it over there, near the schoolhouse. Far enough away so the kids wouldn't be a bother, though."

Several looked out the window and murmured approvingly of the spot selected.

"I'll bring in some white oak," volunteered one. Betty recognized Hank Judkins, from way up Flackey's Branch. She had brought his youngest boy into the world.

"Thanks, Hank." Charlie began writing down the promised lumber: 400 feet of black walnut, 200 of poplar. Someone volunteered two windows, another some nails. Charlie glanced over the list to make sure no needed supplies were forgotten.

"Well, Miss Lester, looks like you'll have your clinic." Charlie smiled as he turned to offer Betty a chance to speak to the group.

Betty's speech was short and simple. Although her British accent sounded curiously out of place compared to the mountain twang of the others, her dedication to them and their families was evident. They might call it "Miss Lester's Clinic," but it would be theirs as well.

Somehow, Betty expected the trees for the lumber to begin appearing the next day, or at least by the next week. But tomorrow is just as good as today in the mountains. Weeks went by. Betty hesitated to speak to anyone about it. After all, she didn't want to be one of those pushy "brought-on" people!

Then one morning as she was riding the trail over Thousandsticks Mountain, she caught up with young Elmer Begley. He was on his mule, and dragging along behind the mule was a tree.

"Where are you going with that?" she asked.

"I'm taking it to the mill. It's for your clinic."

That made Betty's day. She now had a good excuse to remind everyone else of their promised donations.

"You're all behind times," she told them up and down the hollows. "One of the boys has already brought his tree to the mill."

Soon freshly cut trees began to fill the lot by George Osborne's mill. When the supply was complete, a day was set for the sawing. Betty thought she'd go over for the occasion. She started Raven up the now-familiar trail across the mountain. Just as she reached the top, she saw a horseman coming up the trail at a gallop. When he pulled to a halt in front of her, one look at Bob's pale face told her something desperate had happened.

"You've got to come quick, Miss Lester. Osborne's mill blowed up! Hiram's killed! They want you down there right away!"

"You get on down to the hospital for the doctor, Bob," Betty said. "Bring him as soon as you can." Betty urged her horse at top speed down the mountain trail. Thoughts crowded through her mind. She knew Osborne's miller, Hiram Young, well. He might not be dead yet. She had learned that the mountain folk often used the expression "killed" when they meant badly hurt. They usually said "killed dead" if the accident was fatal. But what could she do with the few emergency supplies in her saddlebags? And there were no roads to Osborne's mill. Doctor Kooser would have to come the four miles by horseback over the mountain, just as she was doing.

Reaching the mill she hurried to the house next door, since that was where the people were gathered. Hiram lay on the bed. His face, chest, and arms were badly burned. Blood-matted hair told her there must also be a scalp wound. She cleaned away pieces of torn clothing from the burned areas as gently as she could, although Hiram scarcely seemed aware of her presence. Taking clean dressings from her bag, she covered the scorched skin.

As she turned the patient to dress his side, she noticed the strange angle of his leg. "Must be broken," she thought to herself. "Not much I can do about that."

She straightened up from her task at the bedside. Her eyes met those of Hiram's wife. Silently Edna had been watching everything Betty did. Now she spoke.

"What's going to happen, Miss Lester? Is he goin' to live?"

"I think so, Aunt Edna. But we'll have to wait for the doctor to get here before we can do much else. We really need to get him over to the hospital."

Two hours dragged by as they waited for the doctor. Finally, the barking of the dogs up on the mountain told Betty the doctor must be on his way down the trail.

Dr. Kooser could do little beyond what Betty had already done. He did administer a shot of morphine to ease the pain that Hiram was beginning to feel, but when they tried to persuade Hiram to be taken to the hospital he shook his head. No, he'd be all right at home. Hospitals were places you went to die.

Finally Betty and Dr. Kooser gave up their attempts at persuasion. There was little more they could do. Packing their bags, they headed outside for their horses.

"I'll be back over tomorrow," Betty promised as she mounted Raven. "Be sure to give Hiram plenty of water to drink."

The next day, Hiram was little better. Betty tried again to get him to go to the hospital. No success. But by the following day, he was in such pain his thoughts of the hospital were changing. Maybe he would go. This was just what Betty was waiting for. She went over to see George Osborne. Would he be able to get Hiram over to the hospital?

"Sure, Miss Lester. We'll get the men together, and we'll take him over first thing tomorrow morning. Can you be here about six?"

Betty assured him she could. "By the way, Mr. Osborne, did you ever figure out why the mill exploded?"

"Well, mills can be cantankerous, you know, Miss Lester," George replied. "I kinda think it was because the boiler wasn't full of water when he started the fire, but don't say anything like that to him, will you?"

"No, of course not. I just wondered. I'll see you bright and early tomorrow morning." And Betty was off for the hospital.

Six o'clock the next morning found Betty completing her five-mile ride to Bull Creek. She gave Hiram the shot of morphine ordered by Dr. Kooser. It would be a rough trip over the mountain.

The "mountain ambulance" was waiting outside: a stretcher made from two poles and a coat. Thirty men would take turns as stretcher bearers. Hiram was carefully laid on the "stretcher," and they started off up the steep trail. Four men carried for five minutes. Then they would lower the stretcher to the most level part of the trail, and four more men would take up the burden.

The procession moved quietly up the mountain except for occasional grunts from some of the stretcher bearers. As Betty rode along behind she noted, as she had so often before, the stoicism with which mountain people faced their calamities. Their motto seemed to be the biblical, "The Lord giveth and the Lord taketh away." Not a word of complaint escaped Hiram's lips during the six-hour trip.

"Are we 'most there, Miss Lester?" he asked as Betty stooped to give him a drink during one of the changeovers in stretcher bearers.

"Just a little farther, Uncle Hiram. You've been a really good patient," Betty commended.

At last the hospital came into view. Dr. Kooser and the nursing staff were waiting. Burn patients such as Hiram need around the clock care. The small hospital nursing staff didn't have enough extras to provide the special nursing that he needed, so the district nurses took turns staying with him. Betty was the first to volunteer.

Hiram's wife also stayed with him, quietly watching as the nurses cared for him. It didn't take one of the nurses or the doctor to tell her that Hiram wasn't getting better. Each day he seemed to slip further.

Eight days after Hiram came to the hospital, when Betty came on duty at midnight, she noticed he was much worse. As she sat down by the bedside, Hiram opened his eyes. He had recognized no one for days. But now he spoke clearly to Betty.

"Are you the woman that's building that clinic over thar?"

"Yes, I'm the one," Betty replied.

"Well, when I git well, I'll he'p you build it." The words went straight to Betty's heart. How could she tell him he would not be there to build it?

Within the hour, Hiram's eyes closed in the sleep of death. Betty's eyes were dim with tears as she stepped outside the room to tell Aunt Edna that he was gone. The old woman had sat her silent vigil almost continuously since he came to the hospital. Now Betty and the night supervisor asked her if there was anything they could do for her.

"Children, let me set by the fire awhile."

Each of the nurse's rooms had a fireplace. Soon they had a fire going in Al Logan's room. They made Aunt Edna comfortable in a rocking chair. She lit her pipe and sat quietly rocking before the fire. As she shared her memories of the years spent with Hiram, Betty realized how much she had become a part of these mountain families. She was there when babies were born, and she was there when folks died.

Funerals had to be held quickly in the mountains, for there were no morticians, no embalmers. The mountaineers made their own caskets, simple wooden boxes which the women lined with cloth. It was in just such a box carried by his friends and neighbors that Hiram went back to the small family burying plot on Bull Creek.

"But the Bull Creek Clinic will be his monument," Betty thought. "I'll make sure of that."

Six Babies in Five Nights

The smell of methylated alcohol and disinfectant filled the mountain cabin. Betty looked over the newspaper-covered table. Everything was in order for the coming delivery: cotton, rubber gloves, spirit lamp, cord clamp and ties, scissors, hypodermic syringe and drugs, rubber apron, and five kidney-shaped basins. Always had to have five basins: one for cord ties, one for cotton, one for the dressings, another for instruments, and one for the placenta. Water was already beginning to boil in the lard can suspended over the cooking fire.

Marthie's pains were still five or six minutes apart, so it would probably be a little while yet. Betty tied her cotton apron in place and settled down in a chair to wait. Lute, Marthie's husband, sat in the corner quietly chewing tobacco. Every once in a while a sizzle from one of the logs told Betty that Lute had aimed his tobacco juice well.

"You been up this way long, Miss Lester?" Marthie queried.

"No, I'm just relieving your regular nurse. They sent me up to the Red Bird Hospital a few months ago. That's why you haven't met me before."

"Well, I'm glad you're here, Miss Lester. Don't want you to think I'm not. Just that I kinda wondered."

Marthie lapsed into silence, except for the groans that escaped when the pains lasted especially long. When Betty's examination and timing of the pains indicated that the second stage of labor had begun, she started preparing to deliver the baby. She checked for the first appearance of the baby's head.

24

After two more pains, the head began to crown.

"Hold your breath and push, Marthie. But don't push until I tell you. Just pant in between times." Betty carefully guarded the perineum to prevent the jagged tears that could result from too hasty a delivery.

Ease the head out. Wait for the next pain. Rotate the shoulders, first one, then the other. The baby boy slid easily into Betty's waiting hands. A lusty squall filled the cabin. Betty waited until the cord stopped pulsating before clamping and cutting it. She wrapped the baby up in the layette blanket she had brought and held him up for Lute's inspection.

"Reckon I've got another field hand, haven't I?" Lute smiled with satisfaction.

Marthie's smile and sigh of relief came at the same time. Was the smile for that new baby boy or the fact that the pain was momentarily over? Probably both.

Betty placed her hand on Marthie's abdomen to check the uterus. When it had firmed up, hard as a cricket ball, she was assured there would be no post-partum hemorrhage. In a few minutes, the placenta was delivered. Wrapping it in a newspaper, Betty tossed it on the fire. Marthie counted the times it cracked as it burned, for an old mountain belief said that you would have another baby for every time it cracked. Betty couldn't tell if Marthie was pleased with the prediction of three more children!

Betty's horse, hitched to the fence rail outside, had heard the baby cry. She had learned that that sound meant Betty should be going home soon, and she whinnied impatiently. Betty called out to her that it would be awhile yet. She always had to wait an hour or so to be sure that no complications arose.

Soon enough, she was riding down the rough trail at the head of the Red Bird River. This country was some of the steepest in all the Frontier Nursing Service territory. In fact, the nurse assigned to this district had to have two horses, since one wasn't up to continual riding over the rough trails.

No sooner had Betty arrived back at the hospital and unpacked her bags to clean up the contents than she heard the familiar "Hallo-oo-oo!" outside. Not a gentle call, by any means. It was one she could have recognized in her sleep, she had heard it so many times. Fortunately, there were still a few hours of daylight left. Betty saddled another horse and followed the mountaineer as he rode on ahead.

Four miles and one hour later brought them up Dry Branch to a cabin which appeared to be leaning wearily back against the mountain. The woman inside looked as weary as did her cabin. She was a "multip" (nurse's jargon for multipara, a woman who had had more than one baby), so Betty could expect a quick delivery. There was barely enough time to get the setup prepared before Betty "cotched" a baby boy.

Betty completed the cleanup quickly. As she was ready to go, a boy's face peeked in at the door.

"Has the new baby come yet?" he asked.

"Yes, it has. Would you like to see your new brother?"

The boy came in. He couldn't have been more than four years old. Gravely he inspected the new baby.

"Hit's a boy, hain't it?" he said. He didn't sound satisfied with what he saw.

"Yes, isn't that nice?"

"I'd ruther had a sister. Nurse, do you suppose if you'd wash your saddle bags out real well, you'd bring me a sister next time?"

Laughter echoed throughout the cabin. Betty knew that the mountain children were often told that the nurses brought the babies in their saddle bags, a Kentucky version of the stork story.

"Well, we'll see what we can do about that. Just take good care of this one while you're waiting for your little sister," Betty said. With that she was off for Red Bird Hospital.

The next days and nights merged meaninglessly. Saddle her horse, go for a delivery. Come back, clean up the delivery bags, boil the instruments, do the necessary paper work to record the delivery. One delivery followed another, until she realized she had delivered four babies in as many nights. Something of a record, for rarely did one midwife have that many women due so close together.

She looked over the records Marion Price had left before going on vacation. "What's this? Think there might be twins! Better add another layette just in case."

At midnight, there was the familiar call. Babies have the uncanny ability to arrive in the middle of the night. The blacker the night the better, it seems. This call came from Jude. As she followed him out into the night, she wondered if he knew there might be two additions to his family instead of one.

She called ahead to him. "How many children do you have?"

"Three, not counting this one that's coming," Jude shouted back.

"This one. Guess he doesn't know of Marion's suspicion," Betty thought. "I'll not say anything until I see what happens."

The lamplight within the cabin cast dancing shadows on the wall. Betty's abdominal examination told her Marion's suspicion was correct: there were two babies, and they both seemed to be full size.

Her three years of experience would pay off tonight. Delivering twins was difficult enough when they came early and were smaller. These babies would put her skills to the test.

When Betty first came, Mary Breckinridge had said that she didn't look old enough to know anything about babies, let alone how to deliver them. Within the year Mrs. Breckinridge admitted that Betty had a sixth sense about deliveries. She would need that sixth sense tonight!

Betty snipped the membrane—a procedure that usually helped things along.

"Time for you to push, Hattie. When the next pain comes, hold your breath and push hard," Betty instructed.

A girl baby came first. She held it up for Jude's inspection. She tied the cord and cleaned up the baby while she waited for the next one. With twins, a second baby usually comes within five or six minutes.

She glanced up at Jude. Maybe now was the time to tell him. "There's another baby coming, Jude."

"Anither one? Aw, now, not really!" He looked incredulous. "There's never been twins in our family afore this."

"Well, there's going to be tonight." Betty turned back to the task at hand. Two more pains, and the baby's head appeared.

What a welcome sight! Betty had thought they were both head presentations, but she hadn't been sure about the second baby. Breech presentations, in which the baby came bottom first, always ran the risk of being very difficult deliveries.

A moment later she announced, "It's a boy!"

Now it was Hattie's turn to comment. "Ain't that just grand? A girl and a boy. And I don't even have two names ready!"

"That won't be no trouble at all," Jude rejoined. "We'll just call one Betty and the other one Lester!"

It was not the last time that Betty Lester's name would do double duty for naming mountain children.

Hants

The familiar "hallo-oo-oo" sounded below the window of the nurses' quarters about midnight.

"I'm coming," Betty called out the window. She laced up her riding boots with a practiced hand and reached for the delivery saddlebags. As she headed into the dark night, she realized that the man who had come for her had no mule. He had walked several miles to get her. And his wife was a "multip," which meant the baby would come more quickly.

"I'd better go ahead, Sam. That baby might not wait until you get there."

"All right. Sure you won't need a light?" Sam offered the lantern he was carrying.

"No, a lantern only bothers the horse. Horses can see in the dark, you know. I'll be fine." Betty hurried on toward the horse barn. Her horse was saddled and waiting. Throwing the saddlebags behind the saddle, she mounted Raven quickly.

The mountain trail was pitch black, but Raven picked her way carefully up the steep hillside. When they reached the ridge, Raven, a Tennessee walking horse, could use her rapid pace to cover the ground quickly. But Betty was still worried about not making it in time. She remembered a little-used trail that could serve as a shortcut, if she could just locate it in the dark.

"Just past that tall pine, I think." Betty spoke aloud to Raven. She turned Raven off to the right at the head of the hollow. Soon she heard the waters of a small creek and knew she had found the shortcut. They were in deep woods. Not even the starlight penetrated the thick forest. The going was slow because of the rocks.

Suddenly, Raven halted. She snorted, ears pointed, body rigid, trembling all over. There wasn't a sound. Betty strained all her faculties, trying to figure out what was frightening her horse.

"Come on, Raven, there's nothing out there." Betty spoke more soothingly than she felt. "Come on, girl. Let's go."

Raven shook all over, but she took a tentative step forward, then stopped, waiting. After what seemed like an eternity, she took a few more steps. Betty could just barely make out that they were passing an abandoned cabin beside the trail.

"No one lives there now, Raven. Come on. We've got to get going." Gradually, Betty was able to persuade Raven to go on past the cabin and down the trail. How Betty wished she had taken the proffered lantern, or brought her flashlight!

The trail soon widened, and Betty's fear began to dissipate. She had heard stories of wild animals, even of bad men, in the mountains. But she had come to realize that there weren't any wild animals left in these mountains, and she hadn't met any bad men.

Within the hour, she was riding up in front of Sam's cabin. Throwing the reins across the fence, she dashed inside. On time! The baby hadn't beaten her to it.

In fact, everything was quite calm in the cabin. Sue's friend, following an age-old custom, had come to "set up" with her.

Betty examined Sue and found she would have time to get things ready without too much hurry. She spread out the newspapers, put out the basins and instruments, and checked on the boiling water. She sat down on the only available chair. The light from the fireplace flickered pleasantly in the room. Gone was the fright Betty had felt up on the mountainside.

Then Sue spoke up. "Where's Sam, Miss Lester?"

"Oh, I left him to come on over by himself. I was afraid your baby wouldn't wait until I got here, so I hurried on ahead."

"You come by the holler alone, Miss Lester?" the neighbor asked in an awestruck voice.

"Of course, why not?" Betty waited tensely for the answer.

"Don't you know hits hanted? A man was killed up in thar years ago, and you can hear him moaning. I sure wouldn't go by thar, day or night. And you come through thar by yourself alone!"

"Well, I didn't see anything. But my horse did get spooked up near that old cabin. I had a really hard time getting her to go by it." Betty hadn't meant to say anything about her experience, but found herself telling about Raven's reactions.

"And you didn't see or hear nothing?" Sue queried.

"No, Sue," Betty replied, "not a thing. Raven just stopped."

"Well, hit was thar! Your horse seen it," Sue said.

By daybreak Sam and Sue had their new baby girl, Betty had cleaned things up, and she was ready to start back over the mountain.

"You ain't going back the same way, now are you, Miss Lester?" Sue tried to convince Betty.

"Of course I am. I'm not afraid of hants even if my horse is. Besides, it's daylight now. I'll keep a good lookout," Betty promised.

Even the bright rays of the morning sun didn't reach the haunted cabin site. As Betty approached, she noted that it was gloomy and cold.

"What a dreadful place to put a cabin," she thought. "No wonder they think it's haunted." She shivered as she rode past. This time Raven went right up the trail as if nothing had happened the night before.

"Pooh, there's no such thing as hants!" Betty spoke aloud. But it made a good story to tell when she got back to the hospital.

Dr. Kooser was quick to put her in her place. "Your horse just smelled a varmit! Don't you go believing in hants."

"Well, I thought it was worth a try, don't you think?" Betty found it easy to laugh about it now.

The fact that she really did need a shortcut over the mountain bothered Betty though. The men always kept the regular trail cleaned out, cutting down the overhanging limbs so she could go along safely, even at night. Perhaps they would cut her a shortcut that didn't go down by "hanted hollow."

When she presented the idea to a few of the families on the other side of Thousandsticks, they readily agreed. A day was set for "the working." In the mountains, such workings were the occasion for a picnic, a real get-together. Men, women, and children all came.

After sawing, chopping, and hauling trees for several hours, everyone was ready for the fried chicken. Covered dishes yielded dumplings, beans, cornbread, and salad. Betty's food tastes had definitely changed since the days in England. This food was great!

When the ridge trail was completed, the men dubbed it "Betty's Trail." Quite appropriately, it led to "Betty's Branch," named for some long-ago Betty who had lived in those mountains.

Betty's Trail led over Thousandsticks Mountain. There were various tales of how the mountain came to be named that. Betty's favorite was one handed down from Cherokee Indian days. This area had been their hunting ground, and it was said that when they wanted to build a signal fire, they used a thousand sticks.

Not many weeks after Betty's Trail was finished, she and Dr. Kooser received an emergency night call that necessitated their putting the trail to use. Dr. Kooser's horse took the lead as they started up the mountainside. When they reached the ridge, Betty wondered if the doctor would choose the route down through the haunted hollow. After all, he wasn't afraid of hants! Ever full of mischief, she decided to urge him that direction.

It didn't take much urging. Maybe he didn't realize that was where the hants were supposed to be! They rode on silently for some time.

How much further was it to the head of the hollow? Betty wondered. In daylight it had never seemed this far. Had they passed it already without realizing it?

No! Both horses stopped suddenly. Raven had chosen a steep incline on which to halt and Betty nearly slid up on her horse's neck. Then, without warning, Dr. Kooser's horse whirled around, bumped past Betty and Raven, and tore back up the mountainside. Raven didn't wait for Betty's guidance. She, too, took off on the double. When the mad dash up the hill had ended, Dr. Kooser turned to Betty.

"Whatever happened back there?" he demanded.

"Oh, that's the place that's haunted. I thought you knew."

"Come on, now. Are you sure?" Dr. Kooser was still trying to quiet his horse as he spoke.

"Yes, that's the place. I tried to tell you. I've even heard since then that a man was murdered there, for his money or something, and they threw his body amongst the rocks. His spirit is supposed to moan there ever since," Betty reported.

"Next thing you'll be telling me you believe it when these people tell you not to ride past a graveyard because the hants come out and ride on the back of your horse!" Dr. Kooser snorted.

But Betty noticed that when they turned around to go on to their patient's home, the disbelieving doctor took the regular trail, not the shortcut through the hollow. Probably because he didn't want to frighten his horse! She'd give him the benefit of the doubt.

It wouldn't be hants she'd worry about next time.

No Guns Allowed

Gunshots echoed throughout the valley. Even from the hospital, Betty could hear the distant thud of hoofbeats on the hard-packed dirt road.

"What is going on?" she called as she ran to find "Mac."

"It's just Saturday night in Hyden, my dear," replied Annie MacKinnon, the Scottish nurse who served as hospital director. "That's how the young men celebrate. They don't have much else exciting to do."

"What a way to celebrate! Who are they shooting at?" Betty asked.

"No one. They're just shooting into the air. They ride at breakneck speed through town and shoot as they go. You'll get used to it." Mac went calmly on with her reading.

"I doubt that!" Betty thought. "I'll bet people do get hurt."

Her prediction was fulfilled a few weeks later.

"Come quick! There's been a shooting up on Hurricane, and everybody's killed," shouted a voice at the hospital door. Two nurses scurried to respond. The man at the barn, anticipating their need when he saw the messenger dash by, had their horses saddled and ready. The dark night closed about them as Betty and Dorothy rode up the Hurricane Creek trail.

Pushing their horses at top speed over the rough trail, they followed the bobbing lantern of the man who had come for them. He was a stranger to them, but no matter. They weren't worried. The shooting was probably over by now.

Rounding a sharp curve in the trail, they came upon a

ghastly scene. By the light of the lantern they could see men lying in the trail, on the bank—everywhere.

How many were there? Which ones were hurt the worst? For that matter, were there any still alive?

Betty and Dorothy set about to do the best inspection they could under the circumstances. Between the one flashlight they had brought and the lantern in the hand of the man who had led them there, they began to assess the extent of the injuries.

Betty knelt beside one man, checking for breathing. A pool of blood soaked the ground beside him. Betty turned him over gently. There was a bubbling sound as she did so. "A chest wound, a punctured lung," she thought. Hastily she pulled some dressings from her emergency saddle bags. The lantern-holder helped her wrap the cloth to hold the dressings in place. The bleeding slowed. The sucking and bubbling sounds ceased. That was all she could do for him right now.

"How are you coming, Dorothy?" Betty's voice broke the still-ness. Until then they had both been working virtually without a sound.

"This one's got a nasty wound in his thigh. I'm not going to hunt for the bullet—or bullets—now. I think he'll make it until we can get him to the hospital. How's yours?" Dorothy asked.

"I've got one taken care of. But this man over here, I'm hav-ing trouble seeing where the blood is coming from," Betty said. "I wonder if anyone's gone for stretcher-bearers. We're going to need all we can get."

"Yes, ma'am," the lantern-holder said. "Clem's got the word out. They'll be coming right soon.

Men began to gather as Betty and Dorothy kept patching and bandaging. Each would survey the scene silently for a few mo-ments, then set to work cutting the necessary poles for a "mountain ambulance."

"There, that one's ready to go." Betty straightened up as the men stepped forward to lift him onto the makeshift stretcher.

"How many have we got?" one of the men asked. Betty hadn't even stopped long enough to count the number of victims.

"There are only three," Dorothy said. "It sure seemed like lots more than that when we first got here!"

"Are you sure we've got them all?" Betty asked.

"I think so." Dorothy shone the beam of her flashlight in the area surrounding the trail. The heavy foliage made it difficult to be sure. It did appear, though, that the shooting had taken place right in the trail.

As each of the wounded men was placed on a stretcher, his bearers started off down the steep mountain trail. Fortunately, the bearers had brought lanterns with them. When Betty and Dorothy had supervised the loading of the last man, they followed the curious procession down the mountain. They could see the light from the lanterns as the men picked their way along.

"That was really a bad one," Betty said.

"I'll say it was. I wonder what caused all that shooting?" Dorothy answered.

"I'll bet it was over moonshine. Probably a still somewhere around," Betty said.

"Shhh. Don't say anything about that. You know Mrs. Breckinridge's instructions. 'Hear nothing, see nothing, say nothing!' where moonshine is concerned," Dorothy reminded Betty.

"Yes, I know. I'll not say any more. But I'd still like to know!" Betty couldn't help but be curious. The prohibition era was at its height in the United States, and Mrs. Breckinridge had no intention of allowing her nurses to get mixed up in law enforcement or to come between mountaineers and federal agents. If the nurses learned anything they were to keep mum about it. She was not afraid of the mountain men. They looked after their nurses. But the bootleggers were another thing.

Betty recalled an incident one of the nurses had related when she first arrived in Kentucky. The nurse was traveling an unfamiliar mountain path when a man stepped out onto the trail and asked her where she was going. She replied by naming the home to which she was headed.

"Then don't get off the path. Just go straight on through," he warned her.

When she got up on the path a ways, she heard three shots. A signal? She figured there must have been a still somewhere around there. The men operating it probably did not know her, so her benefactor protected her by telling her to go straight on, then giving a signal when she had passed.

"These men must not have been treated the same way," Betty thought. "Or they ignored the signal!"

It took several weeks of hospital care, but all of the men lived.

Payment for hospital or midwifery care came in all kinds of things: quilted "kivvers," homemade cane-bottom chairs, eggs, garden produce, or in donated labor to mend fences or whitewash barns. Cash money was very scarce, even though the charge for routine care was only one dollar per year and five dollars for a delivery!

During the time Betty was posted to the hospital at Redbird one of the men volunteered to pay his bill with a gun—a 32-special.

"Just the ticket," Betty thought. "Now I'll have protection when I need it." She accepted the gun as payment.

Betty realized she wasn't much of a shot, so when the neighborhood boys gathered to target practice with the walnuts in the trees on the hospital property she occasionally joined them.

"Want to try, Miss Lester?" one of the boys offered.

"Sure, why not? Now that I've got my own gun, I really ought to practice a bit." Betty took the proffered gun.

Carefully she took aim. Then she shut her eyes and fired. No walnut fell. The bullet hadn't even gone near the tree!

The boys quickly learned about Betty's shooting. Thereafter, they ran to get behind her when she shot. It wasn't safe to be anywhere else!

News of Betty's new gun reached Gladys Peacock's ears. The district supervisor was not happy with that news. On her next visit she made it amply clear. "We don't have guns. That's all there is to it. None of Mrs. Breckinridge's nurses carry guns," Peacock explained. "That's one of the few rules we have, but it's a firm one.

"I understand. Probably wouldn't have done me much good anyway. I couldn't hit a thing with it." Betty got rid of the gun.

She learned her lesson well. Years later, when she was serving as hospital superintendent at Hyden, one of the night watchmen thought it would be a good idea if he carried a gun to handle some rowdies who occasionally hung around the hospital. When Betty found out about it, she told him firmly, "No guns allowed. Those fellows will leave if we ask them. Even if some of them are drunk, there's usually one or two who can persuade the others to leave. The service just doesn't allow guns!"

Only once were any of the nurses fired upon. Ruth, the nurse stationed at Flat Creek, heard someone outside the door of the center one Saturday night. She stepped onto the porch and looked around. No one seemed to be there.

Just then, the beam of her flashlight revealed a man crouching on the ground. His head was bent over. She could see a revolver in his hand.

Ruth hurried back into the house and slammed the door. A shot came through the door, barely missing her. Crash! another shot shattered the mirror.

Ruth and her housemate, Irma, ducked to the floor as the shots kept coming. Six shots in all. Then silence. Silence for a long time. Was he reloading? Had he left? They dared not go outside to find out, and there was no telephone with which to call for help.

It was a long night. The morning sunlight dispelled the fear of the night. Ruth gathered her courage to go outside. The center seemed deserted that Sunday morning. Whoever the man was, he had gone now.

She rode the long miles to Wendover to report. Mrs. Breckinridge sent word to the Clay County sheriff, for the Flat Creek Center was in his territory. The volunteer members of the advisory committee for the center called a committee meeting that evening. All eighteen members expressed their concern over the incident and eagerly offered to help.

The sheriff arrested several men on suspicion, but each was released on bond. One of them told the sheriff, "You know I wouldn't harm them nurses. They helped me raise my children."

It was out of character for any normal mountaineer, drunk or sober, to shoot at any woman, let alone one of the nurses. The consensus was that the shooting could have been done only by someone who was mentally disturbed. Such turned out to be the case. The man was eventually apprehended and taken for treatment.

The mountain men protected their nurses. Mrs. Breckinridge was right. No guns were allowed—or needed.

Floodtides

A rumble of thunder echoed through the hills. Flashes of lightning announced the arrival of a storm. Rain began pelting the roof with a steady drumbeat. Betty rose from her bed and looked out the window. In the flash from a streak of lightning she saw two men hurrying toward the hospital. Quickly she slipped on a housecoat and hurried down the hall toward the front door.

"Bill Morgan!" she exclaimed as the first man stepped inside, dripping water onto the floor. The second man followed.

"You gotta hurry," Bill said.

Betty lit a lantern and went down the hall to waken Edith Batten, the district nurse for Wendover. "Bill Morgan and his brother just came," she said. "It's a terrible night. I hate to send you out in weather like this. I'll go saddle Snip for you."

Betty started for the barn. The roar of the Middle Fork told her that a "tide," as the mountain folk called a flood, was in the making. No horse for Edith tonight, she decided. The nurse would have to cross the river in the boat with the men. She returned to the hospital and talked to the men as they waited for Edith to finish dressing.

"It's the biggest tide ever," Betty said when Edith entered the room a few minutes later. "Mr. Morgan says even the roads are flooded. They'll take you across the river in a boat."

The men glanced nervously at the floor for a minute, then moved toward the door. Edith followed them. Bill opened the door and his brother stepped aside. Edith hesitated a second, then stepped onto the porch that was flooded with water in spite of the roof overhead. She turned and let the two men pass by to lead the way. Betty was closing the door. "Good luck!" she called just before the door shut.

Edith was excited. What could be more thrilling than setting out at three o'clock in the morning with one man carrying the saddlebags over his shoulder, the other the baby's bundle, and she, Edith, bringing up the rear, floundering knee-deep in water as she walked down what had been a road just yesterday.

The little procession came to the boat and halted.

"How heavy are you, Miss Batten?" Bill asked.

What a question in the middle of the night! Edith acknowledged her 165 pounds, though what that had to do with the situation she could not fathom. However, she soon realized that she was not just satisfying idle curiosity. The men needed that information before assigning her a seat in the boat. It was a crudely built craft, about twelve feet long, perhaps two and a half feet wide, and certainly not more than twelve inches deep. The men took their places at either end, though she could scarcely see them in the inky blackness.

The shuddering vibrations as the full force of the current hit the boat told her they must be moving across the river. Edith knew the river. She had crossed it many times on horseback, but it had never seemed so wide before!

Finally, thud! The boat hit the opposite bank. Edith was told to climb out, but she missed her footing and found herself being hauled up from the river by two strong arms. Luckily she had fallen in a shallow part of the river. She heard an animal snort as she stepped onto the river bank.

"Here's our mule," Bill told her. "He'll take you up to our place. He knows the way. We'll follow quick as we can."

Edith had never ridden a mule before, and now she would have to ride one in this crashing thunderstorm all alone. But she climbed on, and Bill gave the mule a slap to start him on his way.

"Remember, Miss Batten, it's to be a boy!" he called after her as the mule started up the hill.

The old mule knew his directions. Edith had to trust him,

because she could recognize nothing. The rain lashed at them, threatening to wash them both down the mountainside. She rode through the dark for what seemed an eternity.

Nora, Bill's wife, seemed very glad to see Edith when she arrived. And in less than an hour, Bill had his first son. Bill arrived at the house just in time to welcome him. He already had three girls. This son was the field hand he wanted. He whistled as he went out to kill a chicken and dress it for the nurse's breakfast.

They still faced the return trip. Looking at the river in daylight, Edith was glad she hadn't been able to see it on their first crossing during the night! She shivered as she stepped in. The water was racing by. The boat looked more frail than ever. It leaked so badly that it kept one man busy bailing while the other pulled for his life across the current.

Edith sat terrified, gripping the sides of the boat. Her fingertips touched the water, for it was that low in the current. The crossing seemed to take hours, though it only took a few minutes. She was glad to get back to the hospital and be able to tell the others of her night's adventures.

That evening, as Edith came into the dining room to join the nurses for dinner, Betty said, "Isn't it too bad about that girl who drowned?"

"Who? Was it someone I know?" Edith asked.

"Annie Fields. From up on Hurricane." Betty replied.

"Oh no!" Edith cried. "Annie Fields is one of my expectant mothers! What happened?"

"She was trying to cross the river, same place as you did, about noon today. The current was so strong it carried the boat with her and her brother downstream. Struck the rocks," Betty said. "Annie was thrown out of the boat. They found her body just an hour ago. These tides are just terrible."

Edith thought about her nighttime adventure. Same river, same crossing, same boat. The river played a deadly game.

"Remember the time Nancy decided to swim her horse when the river was flooded down at Confluence?" Betty inquired of the oldtimers at the table.

"Yes, with ice in the river and all. Wonder she ever got out alive," said Mac, one of the other nurses at the hospital.

"She lost everything. Saddlebags, saddle, layette. When the girth on the saddle broke, there was no way to stay on the horse," Betty said. "How she ever managed to swim with all those clothes on is beyond me. Raincoat, jacket, sweater—and two pair of boots—her rubber ones over the leather ones."

"Yes," Mac added. "She said she thought she was quite clever by wearing rubber boots and leather ones together. I imagine it's the last time she ever does that."

"Wears two pairs of boots, or swims her horse?" Betty asked.

"Both!" Mac replied drily.

"Well, I know I'll never swim a horse if I can help it. When I first came I thought it would be great fun. But that time I urged the Old Gray Mare where she didn't want to go, and she had to end up swimming, I nearly went down the river with her. When I got back here all soaking wet, Dr. Kooser gave me a lecture three miles long!" Betty recalled.

"So that's why you wouldn't swim your horse when Marvin was here making the film?" Mac asked.

Marvin Breckinridge, cousin of Mary Breckinridge and an accomplished photographer, had been at Hyden the past summer to produce a film on the Frontier Nursing Service. Betty had been one of the star performers. She had willingly gone along with most of Marvin's ideas for shots of "the ideal nurse at work," but she had drawn the line at swimming her horse across the river.

"I carried the torch as I rode off into the night," Betty said. "But I wouldn't swim the river for him. That one time scared me enough to last a lifetime."

Two weeks later, another storm set the creeks to rising a foot an hour. Betty, as district supervisor, was visiting the center at Possum Bend.

"Looks like I'll stay longer than I expected," she said to Nancy O'Neil, one of the nurses at the center.

Just then two men brought a call for help up on Bill's Branch. A young boy had been kicked in the head by a mule and was "bad off." The men shook their heads. "His skull bone's a showin' through," they said. Betty volunteered to go with

Nancy on the call. The two men rode along behind as they started up the trail. It was rough country going up to Bill's Branch, even in good weather. The heavy rains made it treacherous. Dead branches and rubble filled the trail. The rain sluiced down as though they were riding under a rainspout.

Nancy and Betty had both heard tales about the treacherous ford at Bill's Branch. As they approached it, they could see the swirling waters carrying all kinds of debris along.

"Can't cross here much longer," one of the men said. The nurses were appalled at the thought of crossing at all.

Nancy looked at the half-submerged boat at the edge of the ford. "We're supposed to go across in that?" she thought.

Betty followed Nancy's gaze and read her thoughts. "Come on, let's get to bailing," she said. They stooped to assist the men with the task. It seemed like a losing battle. Rainwater was filling the boat nearly as fast as they could throw it out. The men finally indicated it was time to climb in and go.

With vigorous strokes of the stout oak oars, they made it across. Betty could just picture the little boat crashing downstream, dashed to pieces on the rocks.

A mile or so up the trail the men led them through a cornfield to a swinging bridge that crossed a creek. Betty had found swinging bridges, with their floor boards set at several inches apart, difficult to manage the first time she had had to cross one. She had closed her eyes while someone led her across! Suspended from cables, the bridges bobbed up and down with every step, and the side rails were never in the right place to hang on.

But Betty's skill at crossing swinging bridges had increased, and now she stepped confidently on the widely spaced planks, even though her eyes never left the rushing waters beneath the bridge.

Just as she reached the end, she heard a sharp crack behind her.

"Help, Betty. Help me!" Nancy cried.

Betty whirled. A plank had broken beneath Nancy. Her feet and legs dangled in the rushing creek, her body suspended over the water by a rail under each armpit.

Betty hurried back and grasped Nancy's arm with one hand

while she hung onto the side cable with the other. The bridge swayed ominously beneath them.

Although the bridge was only wide enough for one person at a time, the two men managed to maneuver beside Nancy and in due time extricated her from the broken bridge. Betty chalked up another point against swinging bridges in her memory book. She had seen the tides take them away completely, leaving only the cables trailing in the water.

Jack, the injured teenager whom they had come to help, really needed to go to the hospital but there was no chance to get him there now. They'd have to do the best they could. His face and forehead were swollen badly. His blood soaked clothes showed that his nose had bled profusely. He was barely able to speak. Through the torn tissue, his "skull bone" was visible, as the men had announced when they came for the nurses.

Jack never complained as the nurses worked. Not a moan nor a whimper, even though he was badly hurt. In spite of the shock to his system and his loss of blood, his pulse and blood pressure were normal. Nancy cleaned and dressed the scalp wound while Betty gave him an anti-tetanus injection and some pills to ease the pain, as authorized by their medical routine.

Betty and Nancy discussed with the family the possibility of getting Jack down to the hospital. "He really needs stitches in that head wound," Nancy said, but they all knew that the weather would have to give its permission first.

As Nancy and Betty prepared to leave, Nancy said, "I don't want to face that bridge again. Do you suppose there's another way around?"

"Well, let's ask," and Betty put the question to one of the men.

"Sure, but hit's a lot longer," and he described the route to Moseley Bend. What was an extra mile compared to the horrors of a swinging bridge with the floor planks missing? It would be a long time before Betty would cross one willingly, and never again in a tide if she could help it.

Varmints

Mr. McKarren's stories of the varmints had been Betty's introduction to Kentucky. Mr. and Mrs. McKarren, as members of the Lexington Committee which supported the work of the FNS in Hyden, usually met new nurses coming in to work for Mary Breckinridge.

"Bears? Those hills are full of them. And mountain lions too. Just wait until you hear one scream!" Mr. McKarren said. That fine summer evening in 1928, sitting on the porch of the McKarren home in Lexington, Betty had been very gullible. It had taken her quite a while to realize he was teasing her.

There were no large varmints left in the mountains. Bears, wolves, and mountain lions had been hunted off decades earlier. Of course, there were plenty of skunks, opossums, squirrels, raccoons. And snakes! Copperheads and rattlers were common.

"These snakes can climb trees, Miss Lester." Many of the men had told her that.

Tree-climbing snakes? Never. Betty put those comments alongside Mr. McKarren's stories. Fanciful, they were. She'd not fall for those kinds of stories again.

Until one afternoon when she was returning from Bull Creek Clinic. She was sauntering along, talking to Raven as usual. Suddenly, she heard a slithering in the branches overhead. She looked up, searching for the source of the sound.

Plop! A snake fell from the branch, landing on the rump of her horse. The horse leaped forward with a snort. The quick movement dislodged the snake. It fell to the ground and wriggled off the trail. It all happened so fast that Betty had no time to see what kind of a snake it was. But it was a big one, of that she was certain!

Raven needed no urging. Horse and rider were of one mind: get home as quickly as possible. Betty could hardly wait to tell everyone. Snakes did climb trees! The men laughed as she shared her new-found information. They had told her that all along.

Not every nurse in the service was so fortunate in her encounters with snakes. Mary Harry, one of Betty's compatriots from England, was a harum-scarum, always getting lost or into scrapes of one kind or another.

"Accident-prone," Betty decided. It was always she whom MacKinnon was sending out to find "Harry." She had not appreciated having to go off searching for this lost nurse.

One evening she located the object of her search over at Coon Creek. Mary was out by the barn, discussing the condition of the cow with its owner, blithely ignorant of the fact that it was well past the time she had said she'd be back. Betty joined them, seethingly inwardly over this cavalier attitude toward time.

Mary leaned back against the barn wall. "Ow!" she cried. "I've been bitten!"

Sure enough, there was a copperhead, lying on the wall bracing of the barn. Mary had leaned squarely on it.

Betty and the man went into action. He ran for a hoe to kill the snake before it got away. Betty went for the antivenin that all of the nurses carried in their saddlebags.

"Lie down, Harry," She called over her shoulder. "I'm going for the antivenin."

After administering the shot, Betty examined the site of the snakebite. High up in Harry's shoulder. "Good thing I got the antivenin that quickly," she muttered. "A bite that close to the head could have proved fatal."

Mary managed to get by with only a few days of general illness, but the bite itself proved bad. The tissue sloughed away. It was many months before she was able to return to work.

However, Mary was no stranger to serious injury. She still carried an abdomen full of shrapnel from the first world war when she had served as a nurse in France. So the varmints in Kentucky did not stop her—just slowed her down a bit.

Snakes could show up anywhere, and often did. One family told Betty of two snakes in their home. One fell from the rafters onto the table, though fortunately not when the family was eating. The other snake ended its own life rather quickly. It also tumbled down from the rafters and landed in the gravy sizzling on the stove!

Not everyone feared the snakes however. Holiness snake handlers proved their faith by holding poisonous snakes. Often they would quote to Betty the Bible texts supporting their religious beliefs. But she always declined invitations to watch such rituals. She had cared for too many snake handlers who had been badly bitten.

"Snakes can be quite pretty, don't you think?" Rose, one of the new nurses, commented to Betty. "I like to watch them swim in the river when I'm riding by."

"Well, that's fine for you," Betty replied. "Myself, I've never admired them very much. Someone is always offering a set of rattles from a snake he has killed. I never take them!"

"Oh, I would. What a memento that would be to show to my city friends," Rose said.

Rose did not have to wait long for a chance at some rattles. The next week, as she was returning from a call in the late afternoon, she noticed something lying across the road. Approaching close by, she could see that it was a snake. "I'll just ride by and not disturb it," she thought. "But, my, it is an awfully big one." She noted its rather small head, its thick body, and its rattle-tipped tail!

What to do? "Shouldn't leave a dangerous snake to escape," she thought. She looked up the steep bank on one side and down to the river on the other. It might be some time before anyone came by to help her "do it in." She knew the nearest house had only a mother and three small children at home. Besides, if she left to call for help, the snake could easily disappear by the time she returned.

She rode back down the trail a short distance and tied her horse to a tree. As she walked in the direction of the snake, she cast her eyes about for a suitable weapon. There was not a loose limb of any size or strength available, and the rocks were shaly and soft.

She fired a couple medium-sized rocks at the snake. They missed and broke up without disturbing it. The third, however, hit its mark, but only woke the snake up. It coiled, stuck up its tail, and for the first time she heard its whining song as it waved the tip of its tail back and forth. Its little tongue darted out angrily. She threw a larger rock and missed again. The snake coiled behind the rock with the steep bank on either side.

Frantically she climbed the hill, searching for better weapons. In her zeal she got on the far side of the snake. To her horror she saw it begin to slide toward her horse. She realized that the snake, too, was frightened and trying to get away. But if she left it, it would most certainly be in a bad mood for the next person who came along.

She picked up a large stone, all of ten pounds, and pitched it down toward the snake with all her force. It caught the snake on the head, just as it was going over the bank. Its body writhed and twisted. The tail kept singing as she piled on more rocks.

Had she really conquered? The earth was soft where the snake lay. Maybe it wasn't dead yet. She piled on rocks and more rocks. Finally satisfied, she returned to her horse and mounted. A short way down the road she met Kermit, who lived up the road. He was going home for the night.

"I think I've killed a rattlesnake up the road. Would you mind checking it for me?" she asked.

Together they went back to see the snake. Kermit carried a gun, and she knew he could shoot if necessary.

Kermit smiled as he looked at the cairn of rocks she had erected over the snake. He took a stout stick to remove the rocks.

"You've shore killed him," Kermit said. He stretched the snake out and measured its length with a pocket tape. It was forty-two inches long, and it had ten rattles—an old king rattler!

"Hit's skin would make a mighty fine belt," Kermit said. "You want him?"

Rose shivered at the idea of having it so close to her as a belt. "No," she replied, "you can have him if you like."

She even turned down the offer of the rattles. No mementos for Rose or Betty. Snakes would stay etched in their memories forever.

The War in England

In 1939 the long arm of World War II reached deep into the Kentucky hills. Their home country was under attack, and the British nurses felt a strong call to go home to its aid. Annie MacKinnon, "the dour Scotswoman" as Betty called her, urged the nurses to go. One by one, they responded. Even those who were not native Britons volunteered. Gladys Peacock, one of the early builders at the FNS, enrolled as an ambulance driver twenty-four hours after her arrival in London. Peggy Tinline joined a hospital staff in south Devon. Janet Coleman was posted to Worcestershire. Edith and Ethel Mickle ("Mickle Major and Mickle Minor" to the FNS staff) were sent to the Middle East Forces. MacKinnon not only urged the others to go—she went herself and was put in charge of an ambulance train that evacuated the wounded from London.

Betty hesitated long about going. Although she had never taken American citizenship, Kentucky had become more home to her than England. "I couldn't raise my hand and foreswear king and country," she said. But however distant, England was still her country. She would go home to help in its hour of need.

She sailed from New York on the *Georgia*. Since it was a large ship, the government felt that no convoy was needed. But German submarines were no respecters of ships, large or small. There were submarine warnings aplenty. Betty, with her usual aplomb, decided the submarine scares were just that: scares. Nothing would happen. She would make it to England safely.

Only after landing did she learn that the German subs had

indeed chased the *Georgia* and had even fired torpedoes, but all the torpedoes had missed. And Betty was none the wiser until they were safely at anchor up the Mersey River.

She volunteered for civil defense in London, but when the authorities discovered her background in nurse-midwifery they posted her to that duty. She had hoped to stay in London. It was more exciting there. But to the Berkshire Downs country in the west of England she went, and night duty at that.

"Bother! The same old routine I was in years ago," she muttered.

But the night shift at the hospital to which she was assigned turned out to be anything but routine. Wave after wave of German bombers flew low over the Berkshire Downs on their way to Coventry. Betty and the others stood outside to watch them. The next day they learned of the complete devastation the bombers had caused. Victims of the bombing reached every hospital in the area. The war became very real as she tended those broken bodies.

A few months later Betty was sent to London, this time to Mary Abbotts Hospital in Kensington, still in midwifery, still on night duty. This time, however, night duty saved her life. The buzz bombs, Hitler's latest invention, started to fall in London. Horrible things. You could hear them coming. Even during an alert, however, neither hospital staff nor patients went to an underground shelter.

About four o'clock one morning Betty had just sent the girls on her staff to the dining room for a break when the alert sounded. All at once there was a brilliant flash, a terrible explosion, and a blast of air. Everything seemed to be sucked in, then pushed out. She heard the sound of shattering glass, and then there was complete silence.

The hospital must have been hit. But there was still electricity. The lights were still on, although the windows had been darkened for the usual blackout. Betty, her white cap askew, started making rounds of the ward to check on the mothers. Every mother was sitting bolt upright in bed, as if at attention.

"Why are you sitting up?" Betty asked.

"Sister, we can't lie down," a mother replied. "Our beds are full of broken glass."